Bread Machine Cookbook for your Dinner

Cookbook of 50 easy-to-prepare and delicious Bread recipes for your dinner

Raul Wyatt

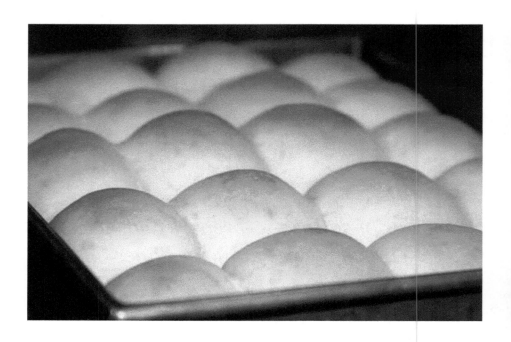

COPYRIGHT

Table of Contents

French Sourdough Bread

Preparation Time: 15 minutes; 1 week (Starter)

2-Pound Loaf

Ingredients:

· 2 cups sourdough starter

· 1 teaspoon salt

· ½ cup water

· 4 cups white bread flour

· 2 tablespoons white cornmeal

Directions:

1.Add ingredients to bread machine pan, saving cornmeal for later.

2.Choose the dough cycle.

3.Conventional Oven:

4.Preheat oven to 375° F.

5.At end of the dough cycle, place dough onto a surface that is floured.

6.Add flour if the dough is sticky.

7.Divide dough into 2 portions and flatten into an oval shape 1½ inch thick.

8.Fold ovals in half lengthwise and pinch seams to elongate.

9.Sprinkle cornmeal onto the baking sheet and place the loaves seam side down.

10. Cover and let rise in until about doubled.

11. Place a deep pan of hot water on the bottom shelf of the oven;

12. Use a knife to make shallow, diagonal slashes in tops of loaves

13. Place the loaves in the oven and sprinkle with a fine water mister. Spray the oven walls as well.

14. Repeat spraying 3 times at one-minute intervals.

15. Remove pan of water after 15 minutes of baking

16. Fully bake for 30 to 40 minutes or until golden brown.

Nutrition:

· Calories: 167

· Carbohydrates: 196 g

· Total Fat: 0.4 g

· Protein: 26.5 g

· Sodium: 240 mg

· Fiber: 7.3 g

Garlic and Herb Flatbread Sourdough

Preparation Time: 1 hour

1½-Pound Loaf

Ingredients:

· Dough

· 1 cup sourdough starter, fed or unfed

· ¾ cup warm water

· 2 teaspoons instant yeast

· 3 cups all-purpose flour

· 1½ teaspoons salt

· 3 tablespoons olive oil

· Topping

· ½ teaspoon dried thyme

· ½ teaspoon dried oregano

· ½ teaspoon dried marjoram

· 1 teaspoon garlic powder

· ¼ teaspoon onion powder

· ¼ teaspoon salt

· ¼ teaspoon pepper

· 3 tablespoons olive oil

Directions:

1.Combine all the dough ingredients in the bowl of a stand mixer, and knead until smooth. Place in a lightly greased bowl and let rise for at least one hour. Punch down, then let rise again for at least one hour.

2.To prepare the topping, mix all ingredients except the olive oil in a small bowl.

3.Lightly grease a 9x13 baking pan or standard baking sheet, and pat and roll the dough into a long rectangle in the pan. Brush the olive oil over the dough, and sprinkle the herb and seasoning mixture over the top. Cover and let rise for 5-10 minutes.

4.Preheat oven to 425° F and bake for 25-30 minutes.

Nutrition:

· Calories: 129

· Fat: 3.7 g

· Protein: 1.1 g

· Sodium: 120 mg

· Carbohydrates: 10 g

Dinner Rolls

Preparation Time: 3 hours

24 Rolls

Ingredients:

· 1 cup sourdough starter

· 1½ cups warm water

· 1 tablespoon yeast

· 1 tablespoon salt

· 2 tablespoons sugar

· 2 tablespoons olive oil

· 5 cups all-purpose flour

· 2 tablespoons butter, melted

Directions:

1.In a large bowl, mix the sourdough starter, water, yeast, salt, sugar, and oil. Add the flour, stirring until the mixture forms a dough. If needed, add more flour. Place the dough in a greased bowl, and let it rise until doubled in size, about 2 hours.

2.Remove the dough from the bowl, and divide it into 2-3inch sized pieces. Place the buns into a greased 9x13 pan, and let them rise, covered, for about an hour.

3.Preheat the oven to 350° F, and bake the rolls for 15 minutes. Remove from the oven, brush with the melted butter, and bake for an additional 5-10 minutes.

Nutrition:

· Calories: 191

· Fat: 2.4 g

· Protein: 3.2 g

· Carbohydrates: 12 g

· Sodium: 240 mg

· Sugar: 1.1 g

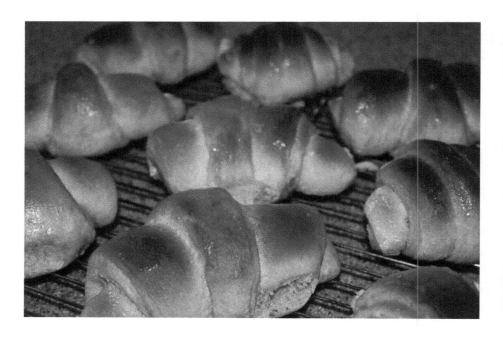

Pumpernickel Bread

Preparation Time: 10 minutes

1½-Pound Loaf

Ingredients:

· 1½ cups warm water

· 1½ tablespoons vegetable oil

· 1/3 cup molasses

· 3 tablespoons cocoa

· 1 tablespoon caraway seed (optional)

· 1½ teaspoons salt

· 1½ cups of bread flour

· 1 cup of rye flour

· 1 cup whole wheat flour

· 1½ tablespoons of vital wheat gluten (optional)

· 2½ teaspoons of bread machine yeast

Directions:

1. Add all ingredients to the bread machine pan

2. Choose the basic bread cycle.

13

3.Take the bread out to cool and enjoy!

Nutrition:

· Calories: 197

· Fat: 1 g

· Carbohydrates: 19 g

· Sodium: 240 mg

· Protein: 3 g

Crusty Sourdough Bread

Preparation Time: 15 minutes

1 week (Starter)

1-Pound Loaf

Ingredients:

· ½ cup water

· 3 cups bread flour

· 2 tablespoons sugar

· 1½ teaspoons salt

· 1 teaspoon bread machine or quick active dry yeast

Directions:

1.Measure 1 cup of starter and remaining bread ingredients, add to bread machine pan.

Choose the basic/white bread cycle with medium or light crust colour

Nutrition:

· Calories: 160

· Carbohydrates: 37 g

· Total Fat: 0 g

· Protein: 5 g

· Sodium: 360 mg

· Fiber: 1 g

Olive and Garlic Sourdough Bread

Preparation Time: 15 minutes

1 week (Starter)

1-Pound Loaf

Ingredients:

· 2 cups sourdough starter

· 1 cup water

· 3 cups flour

· 2 tablespoons olive oil

· 2 tablespoons sugar

· 2 teaspoons salt

· ½ cup chopped black olives

· 6 cloves chopped garlic

Directions:

1.Add starter and bread ingredients to the bread machine pan.

2.Choose the dough cycle.

3.Conventional Oven:

4.Preheat oven to 350° F.

5.When the cycle is complete, if the dough is sticky, add more flour.

6.Shape dough onto a baking sheet or put into a pound pan

7.Bake for 35-45 minutes until golden.

8.Cool before slicing.

Nutrition:

· Calories: 170

· Carbohydrate: 26.5 g

· Total Fat: 0.5 g

· Protein: 3.4 g

· Sodium: 480 mg

· Fiber: 1.1 g

Gluten-Free Bread

Preparation Time: 1 hour

1-Pound Loaf

Ingredients:

· 2 cups rice flour, Potato starch

· 1½ cups Tapioca flour

· ½ cup Xanthan gum

· 2½ teaspoons 2/3 cup powdered milk or ½ non-dairy substitute

· 1½ teaspoons salt

· 3 tablespoons sugar

· 12/3 cups lukewarm water

· 1½ tablespoons dry yeast, granules

· 4 tablespoons butter, melted or margarine

· 1 teaspoon vinegar

· 3 eggs, room temperature

Directions:

1.Add yeast to the bread pan.

2.Add all the flours, Xanthan/ gum, milk powder, salt, and sugar.

3.Beat the eggs, and mix with water, butter, and vinegar.

4. Choose white bread setting at medium or use a 3-4 hours set.

Nutrition:

· Calories: 226

· Fat: 2 g

· Carbohydrates: 29 g

· Protein: 3 g

· Sodium: 360 mg

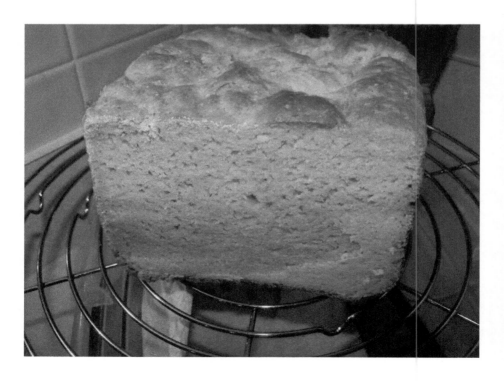

All-Purpose White Bread

Preparation Time: 20 minutes

1-Pound Loaf

Ingredients:

· ¾ cup water

· 1 tablespoon melted butter cooled

· 1 tablespoon sugar

· ¾ teaspoon salt

· 2 tablespoons skim milk powder

· 2 cups white bread flour

· ¾ teaspoon instant yeast

Directions:

1.Add all of the ingredients to your bread machine, carefully following the instructions of the manufacturer.

2.Set the program of your bread machine to Basic/White Bread and set crust type to Medium.

3.Press START.

4.Wait until the cycle completes.

5.Once the pound is ready, take the bucket out and let the pound cool for 5 minutes.

6.Gently shake the bucket to remove the pound.

7.Put to a cooling rack, slice, and serve.

Nutrition:

· Calories: 176

· Fat: 2 g

· Carbohydrates: 27 g

· Protein: 44 g

· Fiber: 2 g

· Sodium: 180 mg

Mustard-flavoured General Bread

Preparation Time: 1 hour

2-Pound Loaf

Ingredients:

· 1¼ cups milk

· 3 tablespoons sunflower milk

· 3 tablespoons sour cream

· 2 tablespoons dry mustard

· 1 whole egg, beaten

· ½ sachet sugar vanilla

· 4 cups flour

· 1 teaspoon dry yeast

· 2 tablespoons sugar

· 2 teaspoons salt

Directions:

1.Take out the bread maker's bucket and pour in milk and sunflower oil, stir and then add sour cream and beaten egg.

2.Add flour, salt, sugar, mustard powder, vanilla sugar, and mix well.

3.Make a small groove in the flour and sprinkle the yeast.

4.Transfer the bucket to your bread maker and cover.

5.Set the program of your bread machine to Basic/White Bread and set crust type to Medium.

6.Press START.

7.Wait until the cycle completes.

8.Once the pound is ready, take the bucket out and let it cool for 5 minutes.

9.Gently shake the bucket to remove the pound.

10. Transfer to a cooling rack, slice, and serve.

Nutrition:

· Calories: 340

· Fat: 5 g

· Carbohydrates: 54 g

· Protein: 5 g

· Fiber: 1 g

· Sodium: 480 mg

Country White Bread

Preparation Time: 20 minutes

1-Pound Loaf

Ingredients:

· 2 teaspoons active dry yeast

· 1½ tablespoons sugar

· 4 cups bread flour

· 1½ teaspoons salt

· 1 large egg

· 1½ tablespoons butter

· 1 cup warm milk, with a temperature of 15 to 115 degrees F (43 to 46 °C)

Directions:

1.Put all the liquid ingredients in the pan. Add all the dry ingredients except the yeast. Use your hand to form a hole in the middle of the dry ingredients. Put the yeast in the spot.

2.Secure the pan in the chamber and close the lid. Choose the basic setting and your preferred crust colour—press start.

3.Once done, transfer the baked bread to a wire rack. Slice once cooled.

Nutrition:

· Calories: 170

· Carbohydrates: 20 g

· Total Fat: 4 g

· Protein: 5 g

Anadama Bread

Preparation Time: 20 minutes

2-Pound Loaf

Ingredients:

· ½ cup sunflower seeds

· 2 teaspoons bread machine yeast

· 4½ cups bread flour

· ¾ cup yellow cornmeal

· 2 tablespoons unsalted butter, cubed

· 1½ teaspoons salt

· ¼ cup dry skim milk powder

· ¼ cup molasses

· 1½ cups water, with a temperature of 1 to 90 degrees F (26 to 32 ⁰C)

Directions:

1.Put all the pan's ingredients, except the sunflower seeds, in this order: water, molasses, milk, salt, butter, cornmeal, flour, and yeast.

2.Put the pan in the machine and cover the lid.

3.Put the sunflower seeds in the fruit and nut dispenser.

4.Turn the machine on and choose the basic setting and your desired colour of the crust—press start.

Nutrition:

· Calories: 170

· Carbohydrates: 25 g

· Total Fat: 2 g

· Protein: 3 g

· Sodium: 360 mg

Apricot Oat

Preparation Time: 1 hour

1-Pound Loaf

Ingredients:

· 4 cups bread flour

· 2/3 cup rolled oats

· 1 tablespoon white sugar

· 2 teaspoons active dry yeast

· 1½ teaspoons salt

· 1 teaspoon ground cinnamon

· 2 tablespoons butter cut up

· 1 2/3 cups orange juice

· ½ cup diced dried apricots

· 2 tablespoons honey, warmed

Directions:

1.Into the bread machine's pan, put the bread ingredients in the order suggested by the manufacturer. Then pour in dried apricots before the knead cycle completes.

2.Immediately remove bread from a machine when it's done and then glaze with warmed honey. Let to cool thoroughly before serving.

Nutrition:

· Calories: 210

· Carbohydrates: 14 g

· Cholesterol: 5 mg

· Total Fat: 2.3 g

· Protein: 1.3 g

· Sodium: 360 mg

Buttermilk White Bread

Preparation Time: 10 minutes

1 ½-Pound Loaf

Ingredients:

· 1½ cups water

· 3 teaspoons honey

· 1 tablespoon margarine

· 1½ teaspoons salt

· 3 cups bread flour

· 2 teaspoons active dry yeast

· 4 teaspoons powdered buttermilk

Directions:

1.Into the bread machine's pan, place the ingredients in the order suggested by the manufacturer: select medium crust and white bread settings. You can use a few yeasts during the hot and humid months of summer.

Nutrition:

· Calories: 240

· Carbohydrate: 5.7 g

· Cholesterol: 1 mg

· Total Fat: 1 g

· Sodium: 360 mg

· Protein: 1 g

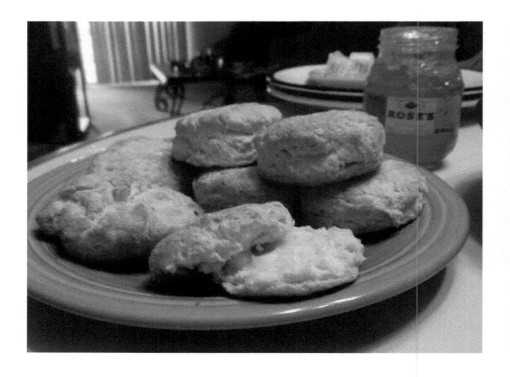

Homemade Wonderful Bread

Preparation Time: 25 minutes

1-Pound Loaf

Ingredients:

· 2½ teaspoons active dry yeast

· ¼ cup warm water

· 1 tablespoon white sugar

· 4 cups all-purpose flour

· ¼ cup dry potato flakes

· ¼ cup dry milk powder

· 2 teaspoons salt

· ¼ cup white sugar

· 2 tablespoons margarine

· 1 cup of warm water (45° C)

Directions:

1.Prepare the yeast, ¼ cup warm water, and sugar to whisk, and then let it sit in 15 minutes.

2.Take all ingredients together with yeast mixture to put in the pan of bread machine according to the manufacturer's recommended order. Choose basic and light crust settings.

Nutrition:

· Calories: 180

· Carbohydrate: 31 g

· Cholesterol: < 1 mg

· Total Fat: 1.1 1/2 g

· Protein: 4.5 g

· Sodium: 480 mg

Honey White Bread

Preparation Time: 10 minutes

1-Pound Loaf

Ingredients:

· 1 cup milk

· 3 tablespoons unsalted butter, melted

· 2 tablespoons honey

· 3 cups bread flour

· ¾ teaspoon salt

· ¾ teaspoon vitamin c powder

· ¾ teaspoon ground ginger

· 1½ teaspoons active dry yeast

Directions:

1.Follow the order as directed in your bread machine manual on how to assemble the ingredients. Use the setting for the Basic Bread cycle.

Nutrition:

· Calories: 172

· Carbohydrates: 21 g

· Cholesterol: 9 mg

· Fat: 3.9 g

· Protein: 5 g

· Sodium: 180 mg

Classic White Bread

Preparation Time: 10 minutes

1½-Pound Loaf

Ingredients:

· ½ cup (15ml) lukewarm whole milk

· 1 cup (25ml) lukewarm water

· 2 tablespoons white sugar

· 1 tablespoon butter, melted

· 1 teaspoon. salt

· 3½ cups (450 g) wheat flour

· 2 tablespoons bread machine yeast

Directions:

1.Place all the dry and liquid ingredients in the pan and follow the instructions for your bread machine.

2.Pay particular attention to measuring the ingredients. Use a cup, measuring spoon, and kitchen scales to do so.

3.Set the baking program to BASIC also set the crust type to MEDIUM.

4.If the dough is too wet, adjust the bread machine and cool for five minutes.

5. Shake the pound out of the pan. If necessary, use a spatula.

6.Wrap the bread with a kitchen towel and set it aside for an hour. Otherwise, you'll calm on a wire rack.

Nutrition:

· Calories: 170

· Total Fat: 2.4 g

· Saturated Fat: 1.2 g

· Cholesterol: 5 g

· Sodium: 160 mg

· Carbohydrates: 46 g

· Dietary Fiber: 2.1 g

· Sugars: 3 g Protein: 7.3 g

Coconut Bran Bread

Preparation Time: 10 minutes

1-Pound Loaf

Ingredients:

· 3¾ cups wheat bread machine / white flour

· 1¾ cups bran meal

· 1¼ cups cream

· 1/3 cup coconut milk

· 2 tablespoons liquid honey

· 2 tablespoons vegetable oil

· 2 teaspoons salt

Directions:

1.Place all the dry and liquid ingredients in the pan and follow the instructions for your bread

2.Pay particular attention to measuring the ingredients. Use a cup, measuring spoon, and kitchen scales to do so.

3.Set the baking program to BASIC also set the crust type to MEDIUM.

4.If the dough is too wet, adjust the bread machine and cool for five minutes.

5.Wrap the bread with a kitchen towel and set it aside for an hour. Otherwise, you'll calm on a wire rack.

Nutrition:

· Calories: 341

· Total Fat: 1½ g

· Saturated Fat: 4.2 g

· Cholesterol: 7g

· Sodium: 480 mg

· Carbohydrate: 59.4 g

· Dietary Fiber: 3.2 g

· Total Sugars: 6.7 g

· Protein:1 g

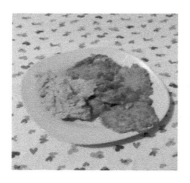

Milk White Bread

Preparation Time: 10 minutes

1½ -Pound Loaf

Ingredients:

· 1¼ cups lukewarm whole milk

· 5¼ cups bread machine wheat flour

· 2 tablespoons butter softened

· 2 tablespoons bread machine yeast

· 1 tablespoons white sugar

· 2 teaspoons salt

Directions:

1.Place all the dry and liquid ingredients in the pan and follow the instructions for your bread machine.

2.Pay particular attention to measuring the ingredients. Use a cup, measuring spoon, and kitchen scales to do so.

3.Set the baking program to primary also set the crust type to medium.

4.If the dough is too wet, adjust the bread machine and cool for five minutes.

5.Shake the pound out of the pan. If necessary, use a spatula.

6.Wrap the bread with a kitchen towel and set it aside for an hour. Otherwise, you'll calm on a wire rack.

Nutrition:

· Calories: 192

· Total fat: 4.5 g

· Saturated fat: 2.4 g

· Cholesterol: 11g

· Sodium: 480 mg

· Carbohydrates: 66.4 g

· Dietary Fiber: 2.4 g

· Sugars: 3.4 g

· Protein:1.1 g

Sour cream wheat bread

Preparation Time: 1 hour

1½-Pound Loaf

Ingredients:

· 1¼ cups lukewarm whole milk

· 5¼ cups wheat bread machine flour

· 2 tablespoons vegetable oil

· 2 tablespoons sour cream

· 2 teaspoons bread machine yeast

· 1 tablespoon white sugar

· 2 teaspoons kosher salt

Directions:

1.Place all the dry and liquid ingredients in the pan and follow the instructions for your bread machine.

2.Pay particular attention to measuring the ingredients. Use a cup, measuring spoon, and kitchen scales to do so.

3.Set the baking program to BASIC also set the crust type to MEDIUM.

4.If the dough is too wet, adjust the bread machine and cool for five minutes.

5.After mixing the dough thoroughly, smear the surface of the merchandise with soured cream.

6.When the program has ended, take the pan out of the bread machine and cool for five minutes.

7.Shake the pound out of the pan. If necessary, use a spatula.

8.Wrap the bread with a kitchen towel and set it aside for an hour or, you can make it cool on a wire rack.

9.Cool, serve, and luxuriate.

Nutrition:

· Calories: 344

· Total Fat: 4.9 g

· Saturated Fat: 1.2 g

· Cholesterol: 1 g

· Sodium: 470 mg

· Carbohydrates: 64.6 g

· Dietary Fiber: 2.4 g

· Total Sugars: 1.7 g

· Protein:1 g

Vanilla Milk Bread

Preparation Time: 15 minutes

2 Pound Loaf

Ingredients:

· 4½ cups wheat bread machine flour

· 1¾ cups lukewarm whole milk

· 1 tablespoon white sugar

· 1 packet vanilla sugar

· 2 tablespoons extra-virgin olive oil

· 2 teaspoons bread machine yeast

· 2 teaspoons sea salt

Directions:

1.Place all the dry and liquid ingredients in the pan and follow the instructions for your bread machine.

2.Pay particular attention to measuring the ingredients. Use a cup, measuring spoon, and kitchen scales to do so.

3.Set, the baking program to BASIC, also set the crust type to MEDIUM.

4.If the dough is too wet, adjust the recipe's flour and liquid quantity.

5.When the program has ended, take the pan out of the bread machine and cool for five minutes.

6.Shake the pound out of the pan. If necessary, use a spatula.

7.Wrap the bread with a kitchen towel and set it aside for an hour. Otherwise, you'll calm on a wire rack.

Nutrition:

· Calories: 221

· Total Fat: 5.7 g

· Saturated Fat: 1.4 g

· Cholesterol: 4 g

· Sodium: 480 mg

· Carbohydrates: 59.1 g

· Dietary Fiber: 2.1 g

· Total Sugars: 4.6 g

· Protein: 9.4 g

Corn Bread

Preparation Time: 1 hour

1-Pound Loaf

Ingredients:

· 3½ cups corn flour

· 1 cup water

· 1½ cups bread machine wheat flour, sifted

· 2 tablespoons butter softened

· ½ cup cornflakes

· 1 tablespoon white sugar

· 2 teaspoons bread machine yeast

· 2 teaspoons Kosher salt

Directions:

1. Place all the dry and liquid ingredients in the pan and follow the instructions for your bread machine.

2. Pay particular attention to measuring the ingredients. Use a cup, measuring spoon, and kitchen scales to do so.

3. Set the baking program to primary also set the crust type to medium.

4. If the dough is too wet, adjust the recipe's flour and liquid quantity.

5. After mixing the dough thoroughly, moisten the merchandise's surface with water and sprinkle with cornflakes.

6. When the program has ended, take the pan out of the bread machine and cool for five minutes.

7. Shake the pound out of the pan. If necessary, use a spatula.

8. Wrap the bread with a kitchen towel and set it aside for an hour. Otherwise, you'll calm on a wire rack.

Nutrition:

· Calories: 319

· Total Fat 5.1 g

· Saturated Fat: 2.1 g

· Cholesterol: 1½ g

· Sodium: 464mg

· Carbohydrates: 62.3 g

· Dietary Fiber 4.11g

· Sugars: 2.1 g

· Protein: 7.3 g

Cream hazelnut bread

Preparation Time: 1 hour

1-Pound Loaf

Ingredients:

· 3½ cups (450 g) wheat bread machine flour

· 1 cup water

· 1¾ cups corn flour

· 5 ounces cream

· 2 tablespoons vegetable oil

· 2 teaspoons bread machine yeast

· 1 tablespoons sugar

· ½ cup hazelnuts, ground

· 2 teaspoons sea salt

Directions:

1.Place all the dry and liquid ingredients in the pan and follow the instructions for your bread machine.

2.Pay particular attention to measuring the ingredients. Use a cup, measuring spoon, and kitchen scales to do so.

3.Set the baking program to BASIC also set the crust type to MEDIUM.

4.If the dough is too wet, adjust the recipe's flour and liquid quantity.

5.After the dough finishes mixing, moisten the merchandise's surface with water and sprinkle with hazelnut.

6.When the program has ended, take the pan out of the bread machine and cool for five minutes.

7.Shake the pound out of the pan. If necessary, use a spatula.

8.Wrap the bread with a kitchen towel and set it aside for an hour. Otherwise, you'll calm on a wire rack.

Nutrition:

· Calories: 405

· Fat: 11 g

· Cholesterol: 13 g

· Sodium: 464 mg

· Carbohydrates: 66.3 g

· Fiber: 4 g

Zucchini Baguettes

Preparation Time: 30 minutes

2 Big Baguettes

Ingredients:

· 5 eggs

· ¾ cup zucchini, finely chopped

· ¾ cup almond flour

· 2 tablespoons. whole psyllium husks

· ½ cup sesame seeds

· ½ teaspoon. salt

· 1½ teaspoons baking powder

Directions:

1.Preheat the oven to 375° F and line a baking sheet with parchment paper.

2.In a bowl, beat eggs with an electric mixer for about 3 minutes. Then add the grated zucchini and fold in thoroughly.

3.In another bowl, mix the dry ingredients, and blend thoroughly into the batter. Allow to rest for 5minutes.

4.Shape 2 big baguettes with wet hands and place on the prepared baking sheet

5. Make 3 decorative cuts across the baguettes.

6.Bake in the middle of the oven for 30 minutes.

7.Cool and serve. Enjoy!

Nutrition:

· Calories: 211

· Fat: 35.4 g

· Protein: 24.9 g

· Carbohydrates: 9 g

· Fiber: 1.2 g

· Sodium: 140 mg

Mediterranean Baguettes

2 Big Baguettes

Preparation Time: 30 minutes

Ingredients:

· 5 eggs

· 10 g feta cheese, mashed

· ¾ cup almond flour

· 1 teaspoon salt

· 2 tablespoons whole psyllium husks

· 2 tablespoons coconut flour

· 2 tablespoons dried Mediterranean oregano

· 1 tablespoon dried thyme

· 1½ teaspoons baking powder

Directions:

1.Preheat the oven to 375° F. Line a baking sheet with parchment paper.

2.In a bowl, beat eggs with a hand mixer. Then fold mashed feta cheese into the batter.

3.In another bowl, mix dry ingredients, then blend thoroughly into the batter. Allow to rest for 5minutes.

4.Shape 2 big baguettes with wet hands and place them on the parchment-lined baking sheet.

5.Bake in the middle of the oven until golden brown, about 30 minutes.

6.Cool and serve. Enjoy

Nutrition:

· Calories: 411

· Fat: 21 g

· Protein: 25 g

· Carbohydrates: 7.4 g

· Sodium: 160 mg

· Fiber: 2.2 mg

Best Bread for kethogenic diet

Preparation Time: 30 minutes

1 Pound Loaf

Ingredients:

· 1½ cups almond flour

· 6 eggs, separated

· ½ cup water

· 4 tablespoons butter, melted

· 3 teaspoons baking powder

· ¼ teaspoon cream of tartar

· 1 pinch pink salt

· 6 drops stevia

Directions:

1.Preheat the oven to 375° F.

2.To the egg whites, add the cream of tartar and beat until soft peaks form.

3.In a food processor, add the salt, baking powder, almond flour, melted butter, and 1/3 of the beaten egg whites.

4.Mix until combined.

5.Add the remaining egg whites and process to mix. Don't over mix.

6.Pour in prepared 1½ x 4 pound pan.

7. Bake for 30 minutes.

Serve and enjoy!

Nutrition:

· Calories: 190

· Fat: 7 g

· Protein: 3 g

· Carbohydrates: 2 g

· Fiber: 1.5 g

· Sodium: 30 mg

Microwave Bread for keto diet

Preparation Time: 5 minutes

1-Pound Loaf

Ingredients:

· 3 tablespoons almond flour

· 1 egg

· 1 pinch salt

· ½ cup water

· 1 tablespoon butter

· ½ teaspoon baking powder

Directions:

1.Melt butter in the microwave in a bowl.

2.Add the egg, baking powder, and almond flour to the butter Beat to mix well.

3.Microwave for 90 seconds.

4.Release from the bowl.

5.Slice in half and toast in the toaster. Serve and enjoy!

Nutrition:

· Calories: 190

· Fat: 21 g

· Protein: 4 g

· Carbohydrates: 4 g

· Fiber: 1.7 g

· Sodium: 30 mg

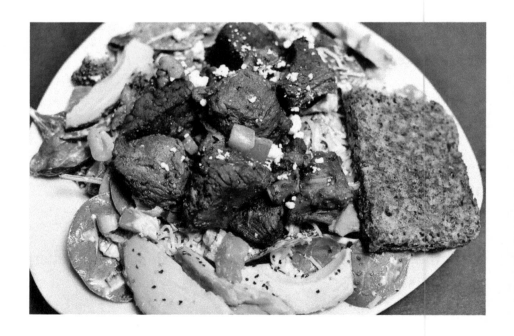

Cinnamon Bread

2-Pound Loaf

Preparation Time: 30 minutes

Ingredients:

· 3 eggs

· 1 teaspoon vinegar

· 3 tablespoons salted butter

· 2 tablespoons water

· 1 pinch salt

· ½ cup coconut flour

· ½ teaspoon baking soda

· 1 teaspoon cinnamon

· ½ teaspoon baking powder

· 1/3 cup sour cream

· 1½ teaspoons stevia

Direction:

1.Preheat the oven to 350° F.

2. Grease a pound pan and line the bottom with parchment paper.

3.Mix dry ingredients in a bowl and whisk well.

4.Add remaining ingredients to the dry mix and mix well.

5.Taste for sweetness. Adjust seasoning.

6.Let the mix stand for 3 minutes.

7.Spread batter into pound pan and bake for 25 to 30 minutes.

8.Cool and load. Serve and enjoy!

Nutrition:

· Calories: 361

· Fat: 45 g

· Protein: 11 g

· Carbohydrates: 9 g

· Fiber: 2.1 g

· Sodium: 30 mg

Coconut Bread

Preparation Time: 40 minutes

2-Pound Loaf

Ingredients:

· 1½ cups coconut flour

· ¼ teaspoon. baking powder

· 1½ teaspoon salt

· 1 tablespoon coconut oil, melted

· 1 egg

Directions:

1.Preheat the oven to 350° F.

2.Add the coconut flour, baking powder, and salt to a bowl.

3.Add the oil and eggs. Stir to mix.

4.Let the batter sit for several minutes.

5.Pour half the batter into the baking pan.

6.Spread it to form a circle, then repeat with the remaining batter.

7.Bake in the oven for 5minutes.

8.Once the bread has reached a golden brown texture, let it cool and serve. Enjoy!

Nutrition:

· Calories: 297

· Fat: 1 g

· Protein: 15 g

· Carbohydrates: 4 g

· Fiber: 1.6 g

· Sodium: 360 mg

Sandwich Bread

Preparation Time: 45 minutes

1½-Pound Loaf

Ingredients:

· ½ cup sifted coconut flour

· ¼ cup almond flour, sifted

· 6 eggs, whites, and yolks separated

· ½ cup coconut oil

· ¼ teaspoon salt

· 3 tablespoons water

· 1 tablespoon apple cider vinegar

Directions:

1. Preheat the oven to 350° F.

2. Grease a 4-inch-pound pan with oil.

3. Place a piece of parchment paper on the bottom of the pan.

4. Cream coconut oil in a food processor and add egg yolks at a time.

5. Pulse to combine coconut oil and yolks.

6.Add sifted coconut and almond flour, baking powder, apple cider vinegar, salt, and water to a food processor and pulse until combined.

7.Take a mixing bowl and beat egg whites.

8. Fold in coconut flour. Mix into egg whites and mix.

9.Pour the batter into a prepared pound pan and bake for 40 to 45 minutes.

10. Cover it with aluminum foil, about halfway through

11. Let it cool and then slice. Serve and enjoy!

Nutrition:

· Calories: 250

· Fat: 11 g

· Protein: 5 g

· Carbohydrates: 7 g

· Fiber: 1.2 g

Multi-Purpose Bread for keto diet

Preparation Time: 1 hour 30 minutes

1½-Pound Loaf

Ingredients:

· 6 egg whites

· 2 eggs whole

· 1 cup water

· ½ cup coconut flour

· 1½ cups sesame seed flour

· 1/3 cup psyllium husk powder

· 1 tablespoon baking powder

· ½ teaspoon salt

· 2 cups boiling water

Directions:

1. Preheat the oven to 350° F.

2. Line a pound pan with parchment paper and set aside.

3. Whisk egg whites and whole eggs.

4. Combine dry ingredients and egg mix.

5.Place in a mixer, and combine to make a thick dough.

6.Gradually pour in boiling water and mix well.

7. Transfer mix to prepared pound pan and bake for 90 minutes. Remove and cool. Serve and enjoy!

Nutrition:

· Calories: 350

· Fat: 21 g

· Protein: 17 g

· Carbohydrates: 9 g

· Fiber: 1.1 g

· Sodium: 120 mg

Eggy Coconut Bread

Preparation Time: 40 minutes

2-Pound Loaf

Ingredients:

· 4 eggs

· 1 cup water

· 2 tablespoons apple cider vinegar

· ¼ cup plus 1 teaspoon coconut oil, melted

· ½ teaspoon garlic powder

· ½ cup coconut flour

· ½ teaspoon baking soda

· ¼ tablespoon salt

Directions:

1.Preheat the oven to 350° F.

2.Grease a baking tin with 1 tsp. coconut oil. Set aside.

3.Add eggs to a blender along with vinegar, water, and ¼ cup coconut oil. Blend for 30 seconds.

4.Add coconut flour, baking soda, garlic powder, and salt. Blend for 1 minute.

5.Transfer to the baking tin.

6.Bake for 40 minutes.

Serve and enjoy!

Nutrition:

· Calories: 297

· Fat: 1 g

· Protein: 15 g

· Carbohydrates: 9 g

· Fiber: 3.1 g

· Sodium: 60 mg

Coconut Flatbread

Preparation Time: 5 minutes

1-Pound Loaf

Ingredients:

· 1½ tablespoons coconut flour

· 1 cup water

· ¼ teaspoon baking powder

· 1½ teaspoons salt

· 1 tablespoon coconut oil, melted

· 1 egg

Directions:

1.Preheat the oven to 350° F.

2.In a bowl, add coconut flour, baking powder, and salt.

3.Add eggs and coconut oil and stir well to mix.

4.Let the batter sit for several minutes.

5.Pour half the batter into the baking pan.

6.Spread it to form a circle, then repeat with the remaining batter.

7.Bake in the oven for 5 minutes.

8.Once baked, remove, and cool.

Serve and enjoy!

Nutrition:

· Calories: 297

· Fat: 1 g

· Protein: 15 g

· Carbohydrates: 5 g

· Fiber: 2.9 g

· Sodium: 360 mg

Garlic Bread for keto diet

Preparation Time: 10 minutes

1-Pound Loaf

Ingredients:

· 5 cups almond flour

· 5 tablespoons psyllium husk powder

· 2 teaspoons baking powder

· 2 teaspoons apple cider vinegar

· 1 cup boiling water

· 3 egg whites

· 4 ounces butter

· 1 garlic clove

· 2 tablespoons chopped parsley

· ½ teaspoon salt

Direction:

1.Preheat your oven to 375 degrees Fahrenheit.

2.Mix the almond flour, psyllium husk powder, baking powder, and salt.

3.Boil the water and mix it with the apple cider vinegar and the egg whites.

4.Mix the dry ingredients to the wet ingredients and form the dough.

5. Make 5 buns with the dough and place them on a greased baking sheet.

6.Put the buns to bake in a preheated oven for 40 to 50 minutes or until they turn golden brown.

7.Make the garlic butter by mixing the melted butter, crushed garlic, chopped parsley, and salt.

8.Brush this mixture on the buns and serve. Enjoy!

Nutrition:

· Calories: 230

· Fat: 27 g

· Protein: 12 g

· Carbohydrates: 1 g

· Fiber: 1.2 g

· Sodium: 120 mg

BLT with Oopsie Bread

Preparation Time: 10 minutes

1 Pound Loaf

Ingredients:

· 3 eggs

· ½ cup water

· 4½ ounces cream cheese

· Pinch salt

· ½ tablespoon psyllium husk powder

· ½ teaspoon baking powder

· 1 ½ tablespoons mayonnaise

· 5 ounces bacon

· 2 ounces lettuce

· 1 tomato, sliced

· Few basil

Directions:

1.Preheat your oven at 300 degrees Fahrenheit.

2.Separate the egg yolks and the egg whites.

3.Beat the egg whites with the salt until the soft foaming mixture emerges.

4.Mix the cream cheese with the egg yolks.

5. Now mix in the baking powder and the psyllium husk powder.

6.Now fold the egg whites in the egg yolk mixture.

7.Put the oopsies on a greased baking tray.

8.Put it to bake in a preheated oven for 25 minutes or until they turn golden brown.

9.For the BLT, fry the bacon pieces until they turn crispy.

10. Spread the mayonnaise on the oopsie bread.

11. Now place over the lettuce, sliced tomatoes and chopped basil on top.

12. Finally, put over the fried bacon pieces. Serve and enjoy!

Nutrition:

· Calories: 230

· Fat: 30 g

· Protein: 5 g

· Carbohydrates: 0.5 g

· Fiber: 1 g

· Sodium: 30 mg

Oopsie Bread Rolls

Preparation Time: 40 minutes

1-Pound Loaf

Ingredients:

· 3 eggs

· 1½ teaspoons cream of tartar

· 3 ounces cream cheese

· 1½ teaspoons salt

Directions:

1.Preheat your oven at 300 degrees Fahrenheit.

2.Separate the egg yolks and the egg whites.

3.Whip the egg whites with the cream of tartar until soft peaks form.

4.Now in another bowl mix the egg yolks, cream cheese, and salt.

5.Now fold the egg whites into the egg yolk mixture.

6.Pour the batter into a greased pan and put to bake in a preheated oven for 30 minutes.

7.Cool for a few minutes and then serve. Enjoy!

Nutrition:

· Calories: 255

· Fat: 27 g

· Protein: 5 g

· Carbohydrates: 0.9 g

· Fiber: 1 g

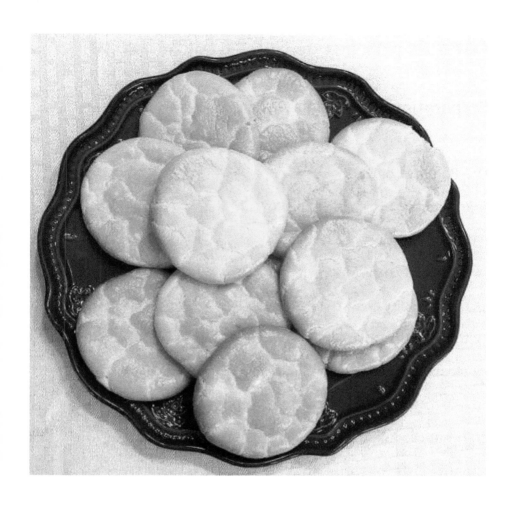

Corn Poppy Seeds Sour Cream Bread

Preparation Time: 1 hour

1½-Pounds Loaf

Ingredients:

· 3½ cups all-purpose flour

· 1¾ cups of corn flour

· 5 ounces sour cream

· 2 tablespoons corn oil

· 2 teaspoons active dry yeast

· 2 teaspoons salt

· 5¼ ounces lukewarm water

· poppy seeds for sprinkling

Directions:

1.Select the program of your bread machine to BASIC and choose the crust colour to MEDIUM.

2.Press START.

3.After the kneading, brush the pound with the water and sprinkle with poppy seeds.

4.Wait until the program completes.

5.When done, take the bucket out and let it cool for 5minutes.

6.Shake the pound from the pan and let cool for 30 minutes on a cooling rack.

7. Slice, serve, and enjoy the taste of fragrant homemade bread.

Nutrition:

· Calories: 223

· Total Fat: 4.1½ g

· Saturated Fat: 1.6 g

· Cholesterol: 4 g

· Sodium: 297 mg

· Carbohydrates: 39.9 g

· Dietary Fiber: 2.6 g

· Total Sugars: 0.2 g

· Protein: 5.2 g

· Vitamin D: 0 mcg

· Calcium:1mg

· Iron: 2 mg

· Potassium: 117 mg

Oatmeal Bread

Preparation Time: 10 minutes

1½-Pound Loaf

Ingredients:

· 1½ teaspoons active dry yeast

· 2 cups white bread flour, sifted

· ½ cup

· oatmeal flour

· 1 teaspoon salt

· 2 tablespoons liquid honey (can be replaced with sugar)

· ½ cup

· yogurt

· 1 tablespoon butter, melted

· ¾ cup

· lukewarm water

· 2 tablespoons oatmeal flakes

Directions:

1.Prepare all of the ingredients for your bread and measuring means (a cup, a spoon, kitchen scales).

2.Carefully measure the ingredients into the pan.

3.Place all of the ingredients into a bread bucket in the right order and follow your bread machine's manual.

4.Close the cover.

5.Select the program of your bread machine to BASIC and choose the crust colour to MEDIUM.

6.Press START.

7.After the kneading, lubricate the pound's surface water or egg yolk and sprinkle with oat flakes.

8.Wait until the program completes.

9.When done, take the bucket out and let it cool for 5-5minutes.

10. Shake the pound from the pan and let cool for 30 minutes on a cooling rack.

11. Slice, serve, and enjoy the taste of fragrant homemade bread.

Nutrition:

· Calories: 176

· Sodium: 240 mg

· Carbohydrate: 32.9 g

· Dietary Fiber: 1.6 g

Simple Dark Rye Bread

Preparation Time: 10 minutes

1-Pound Loaf

Ingredients:

· 2/3 cup lukewarm water

· 1 tablespoon melted butter cooled

· ¼ cup molasses

· ¼ teaspoon salt

· 1 tablespoon unsweetened cocoa powder

· ½ cup rye flour

· pinch of ground nutmeg

· 1¼ cups white wheat flour sifted

· 1 teaspoon active dry yeast

Directions:

1.Prepare all of the ingredients for your bread and measuring means (a cup, a spoon, kitchen scales).

2.Carefully measure the ingredients into the pan.

3.Place all of the ingredients into the bread bucket in the right order and follow your bread machine's manual.

4.Close the cover.

5.Select the program of your bread machine to BASIC and choose the crust colour to MEDIUM.

6. Wait until the program completes.

7.When done, take the bucket out and let it cool for 5 minutes.

8.Shake the pound from the pan and let cool for 30 minutes on a cooling rack.

9.Slice, serve, and enjoy the taste of fragrant homemade bread.

Nutrition:

· Calories: 181

· Total Fat: 2.1 g

· Saturated Fat: 1 g

· Cholesterol: 4 g

· Sodium: 60 mg

· Carbohydrates: 29.4 g

· Sugars: 5.9 g

· Protein: 4.2 g

· Vitamin D: 1 mcg

· Calcium: 30 mg

Walnut Bread

Preparation Time: 10 minutes

1-Pound Loaf

Ingredients:

· 4 cups wheat flour, sifted

· ½ cup lukewarm water

· ½ cup lukewarm milk

· 2 whole eggs

· ½ cup walnuts, fried and chopped

· 1 tablespoon walnut oil

· 1 tablespoon brown sugar

· 1 teaspoon salt

· 1 teaspoon active dry yeast

Directions:

1.Prepare all of the ingredients for your bread and measuring means (a cup, a spoon, kitchen scales).

2.Carefully measure the ingredients into the pan.

3.Place all of the ingredients into the bread bucket in the right order. Follow your manual bread machine.

4.Close the cover.

5.Select your bread machine's program to FRENCH BREAD and choose the crust colour to MEDIUM.

6. Press START.

7.Wait until the program completes.

8.When done, take the bucket out and let it cool for 5minutes.

9.Shake the pound from the pan and let cool for 30 minutes on a cooling rack.

10. Slice, serve, and enjoy the taste of fragrant homemade bread.

Nutrition:

· Calories: 257

· Total Fat: 6.7 g

· Saturated Fat: 1 g

· Cholesterol: 34 g

· Sodium: 242 mg

· Carbohydrate: 40.1 g

· Dietary Fiber: 1.9 g

· Sugars: 2 g

· Protein:1.3 g

Sauerkraut Bread

Preparation Time: 15 minutes

1½-Pound Loaf

Ingredients:

· 1 cup lukewarm water

· ¼ cup cabbage brine

· ½ cup finely chopped cabbage

· 2 tablespoons sunflower oil

· 2 teaspoons white sugar

· 1½ teaspoons salt

· 2 1/3cups rye flour

· 2 1/3cups wheat flour

· 2 teaspoons dry kvass

· 2 teaspoons active dry yeast

Directions:

1.Prepare all of the ingredients for your bread and measuring means (a cup, a spoon, kitchen scales).

2.Finely chop the sauerkraut.

3.Carefully measure the ingredients into the pan.

4.Place all of the ingredients into a bucket in the right order, follow your manual bread machine.

5.Close the cover.

6. Select the program of your bread machine to BASIC and choose the crust colour to DARK.

7.Press START.

8.Wait until the program completes.

9.When done, take the bucket out and let it cool for 5-5minutes.

10. Shake the pound from the pan and let cool for 30 minutes on a cooling rack.

11. Slice, serve, and enjoy the taste of fragrant homemade bread.

Nutrition:

· Calories: 297

· Total Fat: 4.9 g

· Saturated Fat: 0.5 g

· Cholesterol: 0 g

· Sodium: 360 mg

· Carbohydrates: 55.5 g

· Dietary Fiber: 9.7 g

· Sugars: 1.6 g

Rice Bread

Preparation Time: 10 minutes

2-Pounds Loaf

Ingredients:

· 4½ cups all-purpose flour

· 1 cup of rice, cooked

· 1 cup water

· 1 whole egg, beaten

· 2 tablespoons of milk powder

· 2 teaspoons active dry yeast

· 2 tablespoons butter, melted

· 1 tablespoon sugar

· 2 teaspoons salt

· 1¼ cups lukewarm water

Directions:

1.Prepare all of the ingredients for your bread and measuring means (a cup, a spoon, kitchen scales).

2.Carefully measure the ingredients into the pan.

3.Place all of the ingredients into a bread bucket in the right order, follow your manual bread machine.

4.Close the cover.

5.Select the program of your bread machine to BASIC and choose the crust colour to MEDIUM.

6.Press START.

7.Wait until the program completes.

8.When done, take the bucket out and let it cool for 5minutes.

9.Shake the pound from the pan and let cool for 30 minutes on a cooling rack.

10. Slice, serve, and enjoy the taste of fragrant homemade bread.

Nutrition:

· Calories: 197

· Total Fat: 2.1g S

· Saturated Fat: 1.1 g

· Cholesterol:1 g

· Sodium: 481 mg

· Carbohydrates: 37.1 g

· Dietary Fiber: 1.3 g

· Sugars: 1.4g

· Protein: 5.6g

· Vitamin D: 2 mcg

· Calcium: 23 mg

· Iron: 2 mg

· Potassium: 55 mg

Rice Wheat Bread

Preparation Time: 10 minutes

2-Pound Loaf

Ingredients:

· 4½ cups wheat bread flour

· 1 cup water

· 1 cup rice, cooked

· 1 whole egg

· 2 tablespoons soy sauce

· 2 teaspoons active dried yeast

· 2 tablespoons melted butter

· 1 tablespoon brown sugar

· 2 teaspoons kosher salt

Directions:

1.Prepare all of the ingredients for your bread and measuring means (a cup, a spoon, kitchen scales).

2.Carefully measure the ingredients into the pan.

3.Place all of the ingredients into a bucket in the right order. Follow your manual for the bread machine.

4.Close the cover.

5.Select the program of your bread machine to BASIC and choose the crust colour to MEDIUM.

6. Press START.

7.Wait until the program completes.

8.When done, take the bucket out and let it cool for 5minutes.

9.Shake the pound from the pan and let cool for 30 minutes on a cooling rack.

10. Slice, serve, and enjoy the taste of fragrant homemade bread.

Nutrition:

· Calories: 321

· Total Fat: 4.2 g

· Saturated Fat: 2.1 g

· Cholesterol: 21 g

· Sodium:457 mg

· Carbohydrates: 60.4 g

· Dietary Fiber: 2.2 g

· Sugars: 1.4g

· Protein: 9.1 g

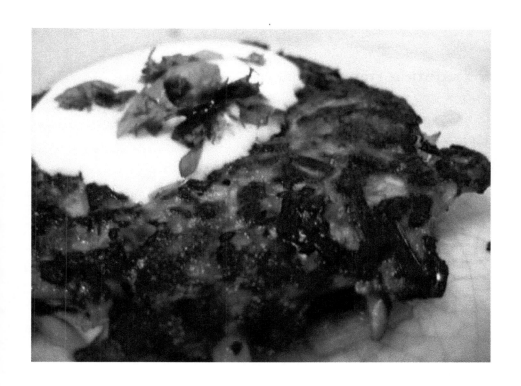

Pepper Bread

Preparation Time: 10 minutes

1-Pound Loaf

Ingredients:

- ¾ cup + 1 tablespoon lukewarm milk
- 3 tablespoons ground red pepper
- 4 teaspoons fresh red pepper, chopped and roasted
- 2 tablespoons butter, melted
- 2 tablespoons brown sugar
- 2/3teaspoon salt
- 2 cups wheat flour
- 1 teaspoon active dry yeast

Directions:

1.Prepare all of the ingredients for your bread and measuring means (a cup, a spoon, kitchen scales).

2.Carefully measure the ingredients into the pan.

3.Place all of the ingredients into a bucket in the right order. Follow your manual for the bread machine.

4.Close the cover.

5.Select the program of your bread machine to BASIC and choose the crust colour to MEDIUM.

6. Press START.

7.Wait until the program completes.

8.When done, take the bucket out and let it cool for 5 minutes.

9.Shake the pound from the pan and let cool for 30 minutes on a cooling rack.

10. Slice, serve, and enjoy the taste of fragrant homemade bread.

Nutrition:

· Calories: 179

· Fat: 4.5 g

· Cholesterol: 5 g

· Sodium: 180 mg

· Carbohydrates: 33 g

· Fiber: 2.3 g

· Sugar: 6.1 g

· Protein: 5.1 g

· Calcium: 43 mg

Crisp White Bread

Preparation Time: 10 minutes

1-pound Loaf

Ingredients:

· ¾ cup lukewarm water

· 1 tablespoon butter, melted

· 1 tablespoon white sugar

· ¾ teaspoon sea salt

· 2 tablespoons of milk powder

· 2 cups wheat flour

· ¾ teaspoon active dry yeast

Directions:

1.Prepare all of the ingredients for your bread and measuring means (a cup, a spoon, kitchen scales).

2.Carefully measure the ingredients into the pan.

3.Put all the ingredients into a bread bucket in the right order, following the manual for your bread machine.

4.Close the cover. Select your bread machine program to BASIC / WHITE BREAD and choose the crust colour to MEDIUM.

5.Press START. Wait until the program completes.

6.When done, take the bucket out and let it cool for 5 minutes.

7. Shake the pound from the pan and let cool for 30 minutes on a cooling rack.

8.Slice and serve.

Nutrition:

· Calories: 183

· Total Fat: 1.4 g

· Saturated Fat: 0.1 g

· Cholesterol: 3 g

· Sodium: 181 mg

· Carbohydrates: 21.6 g

· Dietary Fiber: 0.7 g

· Sugars: 2.1 g

· Protein: 3.3 g

· Calcium: 24 mg

· Potassium: 33 mg

Mediterranean Semolina Bread

Preparation Time: 10 minutes

1½-Pound Loaf

Ingredients:

· 1 cup lukewarm water

· 1 teaspoon salt

· 2½ tablespoons butter, melted

· 2½ teaspoons white sugar

· 2¼ cups all-purpose flour

· 1/3 cup semolina

· 1½ teaspoons active dry yeast

Directions:

1.Prepare all of the ingredients for your bread and measuring means (a cup, a spoon, kitchen scales).

2.Carefully measure the ingredients into the pan.

3.Put all the ingredients into a bread bucket in the right order. Follow your manual for the bread machine.

4.Close the cover.

5.Select your bread machine's program to ITALIAN BREAD / SANDWICH mode and choose the crust colour to MEDIUM.

6.Press START. Wait until the program completes.

7.When done, take the bucket out and let it cool for 5minutes.

8. Shake the pound from the pan and let cool for 30 minutes on a cooling rack.

9.Slice and serve.

Nutrition:

· Calories: 243

· Total Fat:1.1 g

· Saturated Fat: 4.9 g

· Cholesterol:1 g

· Sodium: 240 mg

· Carbohydrates: 37 g

· Dietary Fiber: 1.5 g

· Total Sugars: 2.1 g

· Protein: 5.3 g

· Calcium: 1¼ mg

· Potassium: 1 mg

Mustard Sour Cream Bread

Preparation Time: 10 minutes

2-Pound Loaf

Ingredients:

· 1¼ cups lukewarm milk

· 3 tablespoons sunflower oil

· 3 tablespoons sour cream

· 2 tablespoons dry mustard

· 1 egg

· ½ sachet sugar vanilla

· 4 cups wheat flour

· 1 teaspoon active dry yeast

· 2 tablespoons white sugar

· 2 teaspoons sea salt

Directions:

1.Prepare all of the ingredients for your bread and measuring means (a cup, a spoon, kitchen scales).

2.Carefully measure the ingredients into the pan.

3.Put all the ingredients into a bread bucket in the right order, follow your manual for the bread machine.

4.Cover it. Select the program of your bread machine to BASIC and choose the crust colour to MEDIUM.

5. Press START. Wait until the program completes.

6.When done, take the bucket out and let it cool for 5 minutes.

7.Shake the pound from the pan and let cool for 30 minutes on a cooling rack.

8.Slice, serve, and enjoy the taste of fragrant homemade bread.

Nutrition:

· Calories: 340

· Total Fat: 9.2 g

· Saturated Fat: 1.9 g

· Cholesterol: 26 g

· Sodium: 471 mg

· Carbohydrates: 54.6 g

· Dietary Fiber: 2.2 g

· Sugars: 5.5

· Protein: 9.3 g

Honey Rye Bread

Preparation Time: 10 minutes

1½-Pound Loaf

Ingredients:

· 2¼ cups wheat flour

· ¼ cup rye flour

· 1 cup 10 ml lukewarm water

· 1 egg

· 1 tablespoon olive oil

· 1 teaspoon salt

· 1½ tablespoons liquid honey

· 1 teaspoon active dry yeast

Directions:

1.Prepare all of the ingredients for your bread and measuring means (a cup, a spoon, kitchen scales).

2.Carefully measure the ingredients into the pan.

3.Put all the ingredients into a bread bucket in the right order. Follow your manual for the

4.Close the cover. Select your bread machine program to BASIC and choose the crust colour to MEDIUM or DARK.

5.Press START. Wait until the program completes.

6.When done, take the bucket out and let it cool for 5 minutes.

7.Shake the pound from the pan and let cool for 30 minutes on a cooling rack.

8.Slice, serve, and enjoy the taste of fragrant homemade bread.

Nutrition:

· Calories: 177

· Total Fat: 2.7 g

· Saturated Fat: 0.6 g

· Cholesterol:1 g S

· Sodium: 240 mg

· Carbohydrates: 33.1 g

· Dietary Fiber: 2.0 g

· Sugars: 3.4 g

· Protein: 5.1

Tomato Paprika Bread

Preparation Time: 10 minutes

1½-Pounds Loaf

Ingredients:

· 1½ teaspoons active dry yeast

· 3 cups bread flour

· 2 tablespoons white sugar

· 1 teaspoon salt

· 1½ tablespoons butter, melted

· 1 cup lukewarm water

· 2 teaspoons ground paprika

· 1 cup dried tomatoes, chopped

Directions:

1.Prepare all of the ingredients for your bread and measuring means (a cup, a spoon, kitchen scales).

2.Carefully measure the ingredients into the pan, except the tomatoes.

3.Put all the ingredients into a bread bucket in the right order. Follow your manual for the bread machine.

4.Close the cover.

5.Select your bread machine program to BASIC and choose the crust colour to MEDIUM or DARK.

6.Press START. After the signal, put the chopped tomatoes into the dough.

7.Wait until the program completes.

8.When done, take the bucket out and let it cool for 5 minutes.

9.Shake the pound from the pan and let cool for 30 minutes on a cooling rack.

10. Slice, serve, and enjoy the taste of fragrant homemade bread.

Nutrition:

· Calories: 183

· Total Fat: 4.2 g

· Saturated Fat: 2.6 g

· Cholesterol: 1¼ g

· Sodium: 245 mg

· Carbohydrates: 10.5 g

· Dietary Fiber: 1.2 g

· Protein: 3.1g

· Sugars: 1.9 g

· Calcium: 7 mg

Bran Bread

Preparation Time: 10 minutes

1-Pound Loaf

Ingredients:

· 2½ cups all-purpose flour, sifted

· 1 whole egg

· ¾ cup bran

· 1 cup lukewarm water

· 1 tablespoon sunflower oil

· 2 teaspoons brown sugar

· 1 teaspoon sea salt

· 1 teaspoon active dry yeast

Directions:

1.Prepare all of the ingredients for your bread and measuring means (a cup, a spoon, kitchen scales).

2.Carefully measure the ingredients into the pan.

3.Put all the ingredients into a bread bucket in the right order. Follow your manual for the bread machine.

4.Close the cover. Select your bread machine's program to FRENCH BREAD and choose the crust colour to MEDIUM.

5.Press START.

6.Wait until the program completes.

7. When done, take the bucket out and let it cool for 5minutes.

8.Slice, serve, and enjoy the taste of fragrant homemade bread.

Nutrition:

· Calories: 307

· Total Fat: 5.1 g

· Saturated Fat: 0.9 g

· Cholesterol: 33 g

· Sodium: 240 mg

· Carbohydrates: 54 g

· Dietary Fiber: 7.9 g

· Total Sugars: 1.1 g

· Protein: 1 ¼ g

Honey Beer Bread

Preparation Time: 10 minutes

1½-Pound Loaf

Ingredients:

· 1 1/6 cups light beer, without foam

· 2 tablespoons of liquid honey

· 1 tablespoon olive oil

· 1 teaspoon sea salt

· 1 teaspoon cumin

· 2¾ cups bread flour

· 1½ teaspoons active dry yeast

Directions:

1.Prepare all of the ingredients for your bread and measuring means (a cup, a spoon, kitchen scales).

2.Carefully measure the ingredients into the pan.

3.Put all ingredients into a bread bucket in the right order, follow your manual for the bread machine.

4.Close the cover. Select the program of your bread machine to BASIC and choose the crust colour to MEDIUM.

5.Press START. Wait until the program completes.

6.When done, take the bucket out and let it cool for 5 minutes.

7.Shake the pound from the pan and let cool for 30 minutes on a cooling rack.

8. Slice, serve, and enjoy the taste of fragrant homemade bread.

Nutrition:

· Calories: 210

· Total Fat 1.6 g

· Saturated Fat: 0.2 g

· Cholesterol: 0 g

· Sodium: 240 mg

· Carbohydrates: 42.3 g

· Dietary Fiber: 1.1 g

· Total Sugars: 2.6 g

· Protein: 5.9 g

· Calcium: 1¼ mg

· Potassium: 91 mg

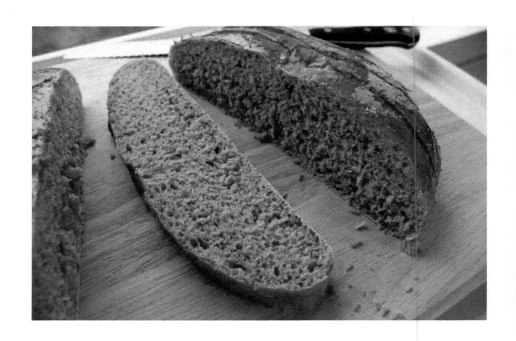

Lightning Source UK Ltd.
Milton Keynes UK
UKHW020803110621
385329UK00001B/92